Contents

3

INTRODUCTION

We are a part of 'The Era of the Lean and Fit'. A glance at any film poster would show lean actors with perfect distribution of body fat in muscular body frames. Let's accept every single person on earth wants to be fit and appear attractive. However, out of the three somatotypes of the human physique, an ectomorph body type is the least favoured of all. Because of less body fat, which in turn is responsible for low body mass index, people with the ectomorph body type often look skinny or even papery. Of all the methods adopted by ectomorphic people to increase body mass, an ectomorph nutritional diet is the best way to increase weight and be fit. If you are an ectomorph, scroll down for weight gain tips through an ectomorph workout and diet plan. Finding the right ectomorph diet is very important since trying to gain weight and muscle mass is the biggest hurdle an ectomorph faces. Known in the bodybuilding world as "hardgainers", these are folks who are not genetically gifted with big muscle-bound bodies, and really have to work hard to see results. However, when those results come they often result in the most sought after, and aesthetically pleasing physiques since the ectomorph has a naturally low body fat percentage.

The trouble is in getting those results. Frustration usually sets in beforehand. Time and again the main reason ectomorphs are not as big as they want to be is simply that they don't eat enough, or they eat the wrong things at the wrong times. What we'll look at here is how we can construct the right ectomorph diet. The success of every bodybuilding program depends on understanding nutrition and diet. And for ectomorph bodybuilders, this is true even more. No doubt, your ectomorph workout is the key, but your ectomorph diet plan is the door behind which lies the strong, muscular body you dream of.

Although for serious ectomorph bodybuilder the diet is important at any time and day, it is the pre-workout and post workout diet plan that has the most immediate impact on your muscles. The nutrients right after your workout will give you a muscle building edge you need in order to progress, while the nutrients you give your body before the workout will have instant effect on the □uality and effectiveness of your training.

You absolutely need to pay a lot of attention to food and supplements you take 90 minutes before and 90 minutes after workout.

Lifting weights not only tires your muscles (and often your mind too), but actually creates a microscopic tears inside your muscles. It is while resting after your training, and especially while sleeping, when your body starts repairing those tears, using the nutrients you provided. Think of the food as the cement that is used to build your muscles.

After workout, your muscles are "hungry", and to feed them quickly and effectively, you should give them fast absorbing carbohydrates, best in the form of glycogen. Without glycogen, your muscles may not be able to start up the recovery process as efficiently as they could with the glycogen.

The best source of glycogen can be found in fruits. I especially like to eat bananas after my workouts, because they are also a great source of potassium.

If you can, instead of eating solid food, consider drinking a post workout supplement. It does not have to be a commercial product, it can be a drink you make yourself, such as fruit juice consisting of various fruits. However, commercial supplement usually has a higher concentration and is more balanced. It may, if considering the actual concentration and ease of preparation be a cheaper option than home made drink.

Either way, it is vitally important you give your body glycogen, no matter how you decide to do it.The second essential nutrient in your post workout diet is, of course, protein. It is protein that is the main building block for your muscles.

You already probably know that the best source of protein is eggs, lean meat or fish, however, these foods take time to be processed and absorbed into your blood stream. Therefore, it is better to actually drink a protein drink after workout. It absorbs □uickly and does not overload your digestive system.

When it comes to post-workout protein, there is no special ectomorph supplement, so the criteria for buying a protein supplement is simply the amount of protein in a serving, and taste and flavor you prefer.

Again, you can mix your own drink, but trust me, the commercial protein drinks are typically actually cheaper when you consider the amount and quality of protein they supply in one serving. Plus, they just taste much better than drinking some milk shake with raw egg whites. Then again, Rocky drank that and it certainly worked for him...

You should take both carbohydrate drink, and protein drink within 30 minutes after workout. Then, 60-90 minutes after workout you should have a regular, □uality meal. The meal should be well balanced carbs and protein meal, such as lean beef or chicken with rice or potatoes.

If you workout at the evening, make sure the meal is not too big. Overeating before going to sleep makes your sleep shallow, and deep sleep is vital for releasing growth hormone and relaxing and building your muscles (remember the little tears in your muscles after the workout that need to be repaired!).

This simple and fairly inexpensive ectomorph diet plan will ensure you give your muscles what they need to grow and get stronger, and you will start seeing dramatic results very soon, even if you are an ectomorph bodybuilder.

If you are one of the thousands of frustrated ectomorph bodybuilders struggling with the same lousy weights day after day, and even lousier results, there is a hope for you!

The good news is, that even you can become muscular and strong. The bad news is, it will be hard and long journey. But if you are ready to put your ectomorph diet plan and workout into higher gear, go to my ectomorph bodybuilder blog where I share tons of great tips specific to ectomorph bodybuilders.

The ectomorph diet can be summed up in this maxim:

Eat Big To Get Big

Eating well and consuming the right amount of calories is the most important part of the ectomorph diet and the biggest stumbling block an ectomorph faces in their workouts and ability to gain mass. The recommended daily calorie intake for an average person is between 2000 - 2500. However, many ectomorphs see this and think that this applies to them too. BIG mistake! Weight gain and weight loss is all about caloric deficits - simply put, to lose weight you need to burn more calories than you consume, and to gain weight you need to consume more calories than you burn. An ectomorph diet of 2500 calories per day is simply not enough to feed your muscles and bulk up quickly. What's worse is that the ectomorph metabolism is usually so fast it works like a furnace constantly burning up calories - if they are not enough calories in your system, your body will start to break down your muscle tissue instead - basically undoing all your hard work. This is the main reason ectomorphs struggle to gain muscle mass even when they train hard.

It obviously depends on factors such as your height, current weight, training regime, and body fat percentage, but the ectomorph diet should consist of anywhere from 3000 calories per day upwards.

People tend to get scared of such high calorie intakes, but they shouldn't be. You see, you need to realise that building muscle is about gaining mass. You can't gain mass if you're on a strict low-calorie diet. What you need is to feed your muscles to gain muscle

mass, and then once you reach your desired size you can change your ectomorph diet to gradually reduce the calorie intake in order to slowly shed the excess body fat - a process known as cutting. This is where the hard work from your workouts really comes to fruition as you become even more defined. The great thing about being an ectomorph is you naturally have a low body fat percentage and find it relatively easy to lose fat.

What's In An Ideal Ectomorph Diet?

While most people (non-ectomorphs) will do best on a diet of 40% carbohydrates, 40% proteins and 20%, an ectomorph diet will be more like 50% carbs, 25 % proteins and 25% good fats.

This should be spread out over 6 meals a day - ideally at 7am, 10am, 12noon, 3pm, 5.30pm and 8.30pm, or something similar.

As an estimate on calorie intake for muscle mass, take your current weight in pounds and multiply it by 22. For example if you weight 150lbs then your rough calorie intake should be around 3300. Please note this is a ballpark figure and depends on many other factors like Quantity of activity, types of foods, your resting metabolic rate etc. Also, please realise that quality of calories is what we want. 3000 calories of Doritos is not sufficient for the ectomorph diet.

Ever wondered how a guy who's a classic ectomorph with horrible genetics managed to pack on over 41 pounds of rock solid muscle in under 6 months and become a champion fitness model and natural bodybuilder? Read Skinny Vinny's story here Ectomorph Diet For Skinny Guys.

Let's look at seven ectomorph-specific weight gain tips that you need to know and abide by.

Tip #1: Do Less In The Gym need to be in the gym

Contrary to what you might think, you should actually do less in the gym if you hope to gain weight. Far too many naturally thin people think that they need to be in the gym six days a week for at least an hour a day.

After all, since they are so thin, this must mean they need to do more to build muscle, right?

Wrong. The problem with this thinking is that it fails to realise that, as a skinny person, you just don't have the same recovery system that the average person does. Remember, muscle is built when you are resting. In the gym, you are actually breaking your muscle tissue down.

So the more time you spend in the gym and the less time you spend resting, the less time you are giving yourself to build that muscle mass.

An ectomorph should limit his gym sessions to 3-4 per week, staying in the gym for 45 minutes or so per session. That's all that's needed to see optimal results.

As you plan these sessions, be sure to focus more on compound movements and exercise, and less on the isolation work that you might be doing right now. You will get more of a hormonal response from the larger compound moves like squats, deadlifts, shoulder press, bench press and rows, which will in turn help you build muscle faster.

If you're too busy doing bicep curls, lateral raises, and leg extensions in the gym to focus on those above mentioned moves, your program is far less effective than it could be.

Tip #2: Track Those Calories

As an ectomorph, you might be putting yourself on a 'see-food' diet. Basically, if you see it, you eat it. In other words, you don't worry about tracking calories. Tracking calories is for those looking for weight loss, you may think.

Wrong. It's just as important for you to track calories as it is for someone who hopes to lose weight. Why? If you don't track calories, you have no way of knowing for sure how many you are getting in.

Most naturally thin people tend to overestimate the number of calories they're consuming, meaning they're not eating nearly as much as they think they are.

In order to see results, an ectomorph needs learn how to increase their calorie intake. If they aren't seeing results, it usually comes down to one simple reason: they aren't eating more calories than they are using.

Tracking calories is a simple and effective way of ensuring you are eating enough calories to see results.

Tip #3: Prioritise Sleep

Prioritise Sleep

The next tip is to prioritise sleep. If you try and get by with six or seven hours of sleep, this could seriously be hindering your success.

Sleep is when your body goes into deep recovery mode and when you can be sure that you are recovering and building muscle. Sleep is also when your body releases growth hormones, which is a key to jumpstarting the rate that you are burning fat.

Aim for eight to nine hours of sleep a night. If building muscle is important to you, you need to find a way to incorporate this into your routine.

Tip #4: Ditch Food With A Low Calorie Density

Food With A Low Calorie Density

As an ectomorph, you will want to avoid foods with a low calorie density.

What do we mean by that? Basically, avoid food that you need to eat a lot of in order to make any significant calorie gains.

A great example of food with a high calorie density is cooked oatmeal. A small serving will give you a big boost of energy and keep you feeling fuller for longer. A quarter cup of oatmeal will contain approximately 80 calories. Since your stomach can only hold so much food, so you will want to focus on getting the best 'bang for your buck', so to speak.

Some great calorie-dense foods include:

Nuts and nut butter

Whey protein powder

Bagels

Dried fruit

Avocados

Salmon

Grass-fed beef

Tip #5: Eat Every Few Hours

Eating little and often is a great way to ensure your body constantly has the fuel it requires.

If you have to eat 4000+ calories per day (which is not uncommon for most ectomorphs), it's far easier to get these calories in by dividing them up into 6-8 meals over the course of the day compared to 3 large, 1000+ calorie meals.

Your stomach simply won't handle that much food that well and you'll be left feeling sluggish for much of the day.

By fueling your body on a continuous basis and eating 400-500 calories per meal, you will keep your energy levels at a consistent level.

Make sure that each meal you eat contains a good levels of lean protein, complex carbohydrates and healthy fats to make it as balanced as possible.

Tip #6: Make Good Use Of Shakes

Make Good Use Of Shakes

Another great way to get your calorie intake up is to make good use of shakes. These are convenient and quick options that will help you hit your daily calorie target. Blending together ingredients means you can up the calorie intake per serving.

Try adding in more calorie dense items into a 'weight gain' shake, such as nut butter, coconut oil, flaxseeds, avocado, cottage cheese, Greek yogurt, or ground up oatmeal.

Do steer clear of commercially prepared weight gainers however. While these may seem like a good idea, as many have 500+ calories per scoop, they are often loaded with sugar and are only going to provide your body with empty calories. They will leave you feeling hungry again □uite □uickly and won't give you the nutrition that you need.

Prepare your own so that you can control exactly what goes into each shake.

Tip #7: Watch Your Extra Activity

Finally, the last tip to remember is to watch your extra activity level. Those who are ectomorphs tend to be rather fidgety in nature, meaning try as they might, they just can't sit still.

They may find that they tend to pace around often, jiggle their foot, or are constantly doing other activities throughout the day because they are so restless.

If this is you, it's time to focus on slowing down. All this extra activity is going to dramatically increase your total daily calorie burn, meaning you will need to eat even more food than you already do to gain weight.

All this extra activity is actually a prominent reason in explaining why many ectomorphs have that particular body type.

If you can relax and slow down a bit, you might come to find that you will achieve your weight gain goals a little easier.

This will take you some time to get rid of this habit as it's something that's been ingrained in you. But, if you can look at your overall daily schedule and try and find ways to relax and take it easy more often, you'll soon get used to it.

So there you have some of the best tips for any ectomorph who is trying to build muscle to know and remember. It's vital that you make some adjustments to how you are living, exercising and eating or you will not see the desired results.

THE ECTOMORPH DIET

HUNTERS CHICKEN

INGREDIENTS

Serves 4

8 skinless chicken thighs

Sea salt and black pepper

8 bay leaves

3 sprigs fresh rosemary

3 cloves of garlic (1 crushed, 2 sliced)

Half a bottle of chianti

Olive oil

6 anchovy fillets

Handful of green or black olives

2 x 400g tins of plum tomatoes

Brown rice to serve

METHOD

Season the chicken with salt and pepper, add crushed garlic, rosemary, bay leaves and cover with the wine. Leave to marinate overnight or at least for an hour.

Preheat your oven to gas mark 4/180 degrees. On the hob heat the sliced garlic until golden in a pan that is big enough for all the ingredients and can also go in the oven. Add the anchovy's, olives, tomatoes (broken up), chicken thighs and the marinade. Bring the mix to the boil and then remove from the heat, cover and place in the oven for 1.5 hours. Skim off any oil that's collected on top and remove the rosemary sprigs and bay leaves. Stir and enjoy! Serve with brown rice, salad or cannellini beans.

DAIRY FREE CARBONARA

CALORIES / MACRONUTRIENTS PER SERVING

Calories Protein Fat Carb

894   58g   31g 86g

INGREDIENTS

Serves 4

4 chicken breasts (chopped)

150g cashew nuts

Paprika (to taste)

200g mushrooms (sliced)

100g pancetta (diced)

Thyme (small bunch)

100ml white wine

400g dried spelt pasta

150ml hot water

400g broccoli

METHOD

Put the water on for your pasta. Saute the pancetta with some thyme and black pepper for 3 minutes and then remove from the pan to a warm plate. Add the chicken, salt, pepper and thyme to the same pan and saute for 4 minutes. Remove the chicken to the warm plate with the pancetta. Add the sliced mushrooms to the pan and saute for 3 minutes. Mix the chicken and pancetta back in and add the white wine, cook for 5 to 7 minutes to reduce the wine. Mix together the hot water, some seasoning, paprika and cashew nuts and blitz to a cream consistency, then add that to your pan and simmer gently. Cook your pasta in your pan of hot water and, once cooked, mix with the chicken and pancetta. Serve with 400g of steamed broccoli.

FLAX SEED AND ALMOND BREAD

CALORIES / MACRONUTRIENTS PER SERVING

Calories Protein Fat Carb

359   11g   30g 4g

METHOD

Mix together the eggs and 3 tablespoons of water. In a separate bowl mix together all the other ingredients with a further 3 tablespoons of water. Then thoroughly mix your wet and dry ingredients before putting in a small loaf tin or tray and baking in the oven at 170 degrees for 30-40 minutes.

* If you prefer you can swap the hazelnuts for 60g of black olives OR 60g of dried cranberries OR some roughly chopped rosemary.

INGREDIENTS

Makes 8 servings of 2 slices each

4 eggs

6 tbsp water

165g dark flax seeds

80g ground almonds

1 tsp baking powder

1 tsp salt

1 tsp caraway seeds

2 tsp honey

1/2 tsp xantham gum

2 tsp poppy seeds

35g sunflower seeds

35g black sesame seeds

20g flaked almonds

90g hazelnuts

FISH AND CHIPS WITH AVOCADO DIP

CALORIES / MACRONUTRIENTS

PER SERVING

Calories Protein Fat Carb

722   37g   37g 62g

METHOD

Pre-heat your oven to 200 degrees. Mix the sweet potato wedges with the rapeseed oil, rosemary sprig, 2 of the garlic cloves and some seasoning. Bake in the oven for 25-30 minutes until crispy. Mix the ☐uinoa, chopped parsley, sesame seeds and some seasoning in a bowl. Whisk the eggs in another bowl. Sieve the flour into another bowl. First coat the cod in the flour, then the eggs and finish in the quinoa mix. Bake in the oven for 12 minutes, or until cooked through. While everything is cooking mix together the avocado, coriander, lemon juice, red pepper flakes and remaining 2 garlic cloves. Blend together until you're happy with the consistency. Serve the fish, chips and avocado dip finished with lemon wedges.

INGREDIENTS

Serves 2

200g cod fillets

100g Quinoa cooked & drained

50g spelt flour

3 eggs

Handful of parsley chopped

10g black sesame seeds

200g sweet potato cut into wedges

Sprig of rosemary

4 cloves of garlic, roughly chopped

2 tbsp rapeseed oil

1 ripe avocado

Handful of coriander, chopped

Juice of 1 lemon

1 tsp red pepper flakes

Lemon wedges for garnish

CHICKEN PESTO AND CASHEWS

CALORIES / MACRONUTRIENTS PER SERVING

Calories Protein Fat Carb

852   48g   43g 80g

METHOD

Puree the cashew nuts with the hot water. Put your pasta on to boil.

Saute the chicken gently for about 3 minutes in the coconut oil. Add the garlic and cherry tomatoes and cook for 5 minutes. Season and add the cashew nut mix and cook for a further 5 minutes. Saute the courgettes in a separate pan so that they caramelise rather than stew. Add the cooked courgettes, the spinach, pine nuts and basil 1 minute before the end. Mix with the cooked pasta and serve.

INGREDIENTS

Serves 2

250g chicken, chopped

75g cashew nuts

150ml hot water

2 cloves garlic, crushed

200g courgettes, diced

120g cherry tomatoes

150g spinach

1 tbsp coconut oil

150g spelt pasta (or other pasta of your choice)

Basil (to taste)

50g pine nuts

CAJUN KEBABS WITH QUINOA SALAD

CALORIES / MACRONUTRIENTS PER SERVING

Calories Protein Fat Carb

429　　37g　18g 32g

METHOD

Preheat your oven to 180 degrees. Chop the chicken and vegetables for the kebabs into large bite sized pieces (leave the prawns whole if you're using them instead of chicken). Mix together all of the ingredients for the cajun spice and then use this to coat all the kebab vegetables and prawns or chicken. Thread onto skewers in any order you like. Bake the kebabs in the oven for 12 minutes, or until the chicken is cooked through. Meanwhile, for the Quinoa salad, cook your quinoa in a small pan (1 part Quinoa to 2 parts cold water with a little salt) bring to the boil and simmer for around 10 minutes. Drain and mix with the other salad ingredients.

INGREDIENTS

Serves 2

250g chicken pieces or large prawns

150g courgette, chopped into chunks

100g mushrooms, chopped into chunks

100g red pepper, chopped into chunks

100g cherry tomatoes

1 red onion, chopped into chunks

Cajun spice

Sprig of thyme

Sprig of rosemary

2 tsp garlic salt

1 tsp onion powder

2 1/2 tsp paprika

1 tsp cayenne pepper

1/2 tsp red pepper flakes

1 tsp black peppercorns

2 tbsp olive oil

Quinoa salad

100g quinoa

100g cucumber, finely diced

Parsley to taste, chopped

1 lemon, juiced

CHICKEN TIKKA

CALORIES / MACRONUTRIENTS PER SERVING

Calories Protein Fat Carb

296   39g   12g 10g

METHOD

Dry saute, grind and sieve the coriander seeds, cinnamon stick, fenugreek seeds, cumin seeds, peppercorns, cloves, nutmeg and bay leaves. If you prefer to use already powdered versions, then add in smaller amounts of each. To this mix, add the rest of the ingredients and then mix with the chicken thighs. Leave to marinate for at least an hour, but ideally overnight. Place on a wire rack with a baking tray underneath. Bake at 180 degrees for 20-25 minutes, or until the chicken is cooked through (try not to overcook!). Finish with a squeeze of lemon and serve with a salad.

INGREDIENTS

Serves 6

900g skinless chicken thighs

Spice mix

4g coriander seeds

15g cinnamon stick

2g fenugreek seeds

6g cumin seeds

6g peppercorns

1g cloves

2g nutmeg

2 bay leaves

5g turmeric

6g paprika

4g red pepper flakes

3 garlic cloves, pureed

15g ginger, pureed

2 lemons, juice only

100g coconut yoghurt

Salt to taste

Salad to serve

CHICKEN CURRY AND RICE

CALORIES / MACRONUTRIENTS PER SERVING

Calories Protein Fat Carb

554   43g   13g 80g

METHOD

Dry saute the cinnamon stick, cardamon pods, peppercorns, coriander seeds, cumin seeds and bay leaves for 4 minutes to release their oils and aroma. Grind together and pass through a sieve. If you prefer to use ready powdered versions just use smaller amounts of each. Add the turmeric, garam masala and paprika. Put to one side. Saute the onions gently for about 10 minutes until they're nicely browned. Add the peppers and saute gently for a further 4 minutes. Add the garlic and ginger purees and cook for 2 minutes. Add the chopped tomatoes and gently simmer for 30-40 minutes.

Let it break down into a sauce. Meanwhile cook the brown rice according to the packet instructions. Once the tomatoes have broken down add the chicken and spice mix. Cook for a further 15 minutes (or until the chicken is cooked through, keep it nice and moist). Serve with the brown rice and finish with a generous handful of chopped coriander and squeeze of lemon. You could also add a little natural yoghurt or coconut milk if you like.

INGREDIENTS

Serves 4

Spice mix

20g cinnamon stick

3g cardamon pods

4g peppercorns

1/2g coriander seeds

2g cumin seeds

2 bay leaves

3g turmeric

2g garam masala

3g paprika

200g onions, chopped or sliced

650g tomatoes, roughly chopped

180g red peppers, chopped

3 cloves of garlic (20g), pureed

20g ginger, pureed

650g skinless chicken thighs

30g tomato puree

200g brown basmati rice

1 lemon, wedges for garnish

Small bunch of coriander, chopped

SPICED CHICKEN ON QUINOA

CALORIES / MACRONUTRIENTS PER SERVING

Calories Protein Fat Carb

360   43g   5g 36g

METHOD

Mix the chicken and marinade ingredients and leave for at least an hour, but ideally overnight. If marinading for an hour, at the same time chop and salt the aubergine for the salad. Remember to rinse the aubergine before using. To make the main dish you need a pan or dish that is large enough to hold all the ingredients and can go in the oven. Cover the bottom of the dish with raw Quinoa. Then add the onions and peppers. Add the thyme and a little salt and pepper. Arrange the marinaded chicken over the top. Finally, pour over the hot stock until the chicken is half covered. Bake for 45 minutes at 180 degrees. Meanwhile, to make the aubergine salad, saute the aubergine for 20 minutes, then add some black pepper, the tomatoes, nutmeg and lemon. Add a little water, bring to the boil and simmer for 25 minutes. Serve with the steamed broccoli.

INGREDIENTS

Serves 6

800g chicken breasts, each cut into 3

Marinade

4 tbsp lemon juice

4 cloves of garlic, crushed

20g ginger, crushed

1 tsp turmeric

1 tsp paprika

1 tsp cumin

1 tsp sumac

1tsp ground cardamon

1 onion, sliced

2 red peppers, sliced

200g raw quinoa

Sprig of thyme

400ml hot chicken stock

600g tender stem broccoli to serve

Warm aubergine salad

1 aubergine (cut & salt 20 mins before)

6 tomatoes, chopped

1 tsp nutmeg

2 tsp lemon juice

MEXICAN CASSEROLE WITH SWEET POTATO

CALORIES / MACRONUTRIENTS PER SERVING

Calories Protein Fat Carb

567   44g   25g 37g

METHOD

Saute the chicken and chorizo for 6 minutes until well sealed. Remove from the pan and pop to one side. In the same pan gently saute the onions and peppers for 10 minutes. Add the garlic and cook for a further 2 minutes. Add the red wine, bring to the boil and reduce so it becomes sticky. Add the tomatoes and tomato puree. Add all the spices and some seasoning and cook for a further 3 minutes. Add the stock, bring to the boil and simmer for 15 minutes. Mix the sliced sweet potatoes with the oregano, garlic salt, black pepper and rapeseed oil. Add the chicken and chorizo back in and pour the entire mix into a casserole dish. Arrange the sliced potato over the top. Bake in the oven at 180 degrees for 20-30 minutes, until the potatoes are crispy and cooked through. Serve with some freshly s□ueezed lime.

INGREDIENTS

Serves 4

100g chorizo, chopped into small cubes

600g skinless chicken thighs deboned

150g onions, roughly chopped

100g red pepper, sliced

100g green pepper, sliced

4 garlic cloves, finely chopped

200ml red wine

400g tomatoes, roughly chopped

3 tsp tomato puree

80g black olives

2 tsp paprika

CLASSIC BOLOGNESE

2 tsp cayenne pepper

1 tsp ground cinnamon

2tsp red pepper flakes

200ml chicken stock

400g sweet potato, washed and sliced

Sprig of oregano

1 tsp garlic salt

Pinch crushed black pepper

2 tbsp rapeseed oil

Lime, cut into wedges for garnish

CALORIES / MACRONUTRIENTS PER SERVING

Calories Protein Fat Carb

555   42g   12g 76g

METHOD

Saute the mince in a little coconut oil and drain in a colander and place to one side. Saute all the vegetables and then add the mince back to the pan and add the passata and tomato puree. Simmer for 30-45 minutes before serving with your choice of wholegrain pasta.

INGREDIENTS

Serves 4

500g beef or pork mince

1 large onion

1 green pepper

2 courgettes

4-5 cloves of garlic

Coconut oil

200g mushrooms

700g jar of passata

2 tbsp tomato puree

300g spelt or wholegrain pasta

These tables let you know if this recipe is suitable for your body-type and goal (Fat loss / Sculpt / Muscle gain). They show whether it's a recipe you can enjoy before or after 5pm as part of your plan and if you need to adapt it slightly by adding or removing carbohydrate.

CHICKEN TRAY BAKE

CALORIES / MACRONUTRIENTS PER SERVING

Calories Protein Fat Carb

665   49g   31g 40g

INGREDIENTS

Serves 2

6 boneless, skinless chicken thighs

1 red pepper, roughly chopped

5 cloves of garlic, roughly chopped

1 courgette, chopped into large chunks

1 red onion, roughly chopped

1 tbsp rapeseed oil

15 cherry tomatoes, left whole

Third of a block of feta, cubed

3-4 handfuls of spinach

400g tin of beans of your choice (mixed, haricot, kidney, borlotti etc)

Salt and pepper

Handful of fresh thyme

2 tsp smoked paprika

Drizzle of balsamic vinegar

METHOD

Preheat the oven to 180 degrees. Put the chicken, red pepper, garlic, courgette, red onion and tomatoes in an oven proof tray and drizzle with the rapeseed oil. Season with the smoked paprika, thyme, salt and pepper. Place in the oven for 25 minutes. Take out the tray and add the tin of beans and put back in the oven for 10 minutes. Then increase the oven temperature to 200 degrees and cook for a further 5 minutes. Take out of the oven and add the feta, spinach and drizzle of balsamic vinegar, mix well so that the feta starts to melt and the spinach wilts.

These tables let you know if this recipe is suitable for your body-type and goal (Fat loss / Sculpt / Muscle gain). They show whether it's a recipe you can enjoy before or after 5pm as part of your plan and if you need to adapt it slightly by adding or removing carbohydrate.

BANANA, CHOCOLATE & NUT BREAD

CALORIES / MACRONUTRIENTS PER SERVING

Calories	Protein	Fat	Carb
285	8g	18g	23g

METHOD

Heat the oven to 180 degrees. Mix together the coconut flour, dark chocolate, almonds, sunflower seeds and baking powder in a mixer. Then add the vanilla essence, bananas (reserve a few slices to decorate the top), eggs and coconut oil and mix again. Once mixed, pour into a lined loaf tin, top with the reserved slices of banana and bake in the oven for 50 to 60 minutes (or until a cake skewer or knife comes out clean). Cool on a rack before turning out of the tin.

INGREDIENTS

Serves 8

60g Coconut flour

100g Dark chocolate

25g Almonds

20g Sunflower seeds

1.5 tsp Baking powder

1 tsp Vanilla essence

4 Large ripe Bananas

4 Medium eggs

3 tbsp Coconut oil

POTATO SALAD WITH ANCHOVY & QUAILS EGG

CALORIES / MACRONUTRIENTS PER SERVING

Calories Protein Fat Carb

95   5g   3g 13g

METHOD

Put the potatoes in a pan of cold water, bring to the boil and simmer until the potatoes are cooked. Once ready, drain in a colander and leave to cool. Meanwhile, bring

30

a medium pan of water to a simmer. Lower the quail eggs into the water and cook for 2 minutes. Lift the □uail eggs out with a slotted spoon and place into cold water. Add the beans to the pan you used for the eggs and simmer for 4 minutes until tender. Remove from the pan with a slotted spoon and plunge into cold water with the eggs. Once the potatoes are ready, peel the eggs and cut them in half. Then, toss the potatoes and beans with the chopped anchovies, herbs, and lemon juice. Then top with the peeled quail eggs and serve.

INGREDIENTS

Serves 2

4 Quails eggs

100g green beans

100g new potatoes, halved or □uartered

1 anchovy, finely chopped

1 tbsp chopped parsley

1 tbsp chopped chives

Juice of half a lemon

These tables let you know if this recipe is suitable for your body-type and goal (Fat loss / Sculpt / Muscle gain). They show whether it's a recipe you can enjoy before or after 5pm as part of your plan and if you need to adapt it slightly by adding or removing carbohydrate.

IMMUNE BOOSTING SMOOTHIE

INGREDIENTS

50g Apricots

Half an Avocado

20g Almonds

50g Berries

Handful of Kale

20g Brazil nuts

30g Watermelon

20g Walnuts

10g Pumpkin seeds

40g Banana

Coconut water

METHOD

Add all of the ingredients to your mixer, top up with coconut water and blend.

AVOID

If you're feeling run down or are concerned about your immune system then it's a good idea to avoid soya and grains. Too many grains, such as rice and Quinoa,

can be harmful because they contain phytates, which bind on to essential nutrients such as zinc and manganese and prevent their absorption. These nutrients are needed to produce powerful antioxidants.

HEART HEALTH SMOOTHIE

INGREDIENTS

100g Berries

Handful of Kale

Handful of Spinach

20g Almonds

10g Sesame seeds

30g Oat bran

10g Pumpkin seeds

Half an avocado

20g Cucumber

20g Apricots

20g Nuts

Probiotic (as pre label)

20g Blackcurrants

20g Strawberries

METHOD

Add all of the ingredients to your mixer, top up with coconut water and blend.

AVOID

If you're concerned about heart health it's a good idea to avoid low fat diets, alcohol, refined foods, grains and artificial fats. Too many grains, such as rice & quinoa, can be harmful because they contain phytates, which bind on to essential nutrients such as zinc and manganese and prevent their absorption. These nutrients are needed to produce powerful antioxidants.

Ingredient Benefit

Berries contain soluble fibre, which lowers cholesterol plus powerful antioxidants that fight free radicals.

Kale & spinach contain fibre and antioxidants and they also lower enzymes that contribute to heart disease.

Almonds & sesame seeds contain calcium required for the action of the heart muscle.

Oat bran, pumpkin seeds & spinach contain magnesium, which is involved with heart muscle contraction and also helps to lower blood pressure.

Avocado, cucumber & apricots contain potassium, which helps to lower blood pressure.

Nuts & avocado contain essential fatty acids which help to thin the blood, plus they're both high in vitamin E, which helps to lower levels of saturated fats. Nuts also contain zinc which is an essential antioxidant.

Spinach helps to lower homocysteine levels. Homocysteine interferes with enzymes that will affect elasten and collagen that will therefore damage arteries. Effectively homosytene affects enzymes that are needed for the integrity of arteries. It also contains folic acid and B6, which help lower homocysteine.

Probiotic help the excretion of cholesterol from the body.

Blackcurrants & strawberries contain vitamin C, which helps to lower cholesterol. They are also powerful antioxidants and help to convert fat into energy, preventing fat build up and atherosclerosis.

Coconut water contains bioactive enzymes that aid digestion, is full of potassium and is also good for a bit of extra flavour.

DETOX SMOOTHIE

INGREDIENTS

50g Beetroot

50g Celery

50g Apple

Handful of Spinach

Spirulina (as per label)

Chlorella (as per label)

30g Carrots

40g Citrus fruits

Cold green tea

METHOD

Add all of the ingredients to your mixer, top up with cold green tea and blend.

AVOID

If you're trying to cleanse your system it's a good idea to avoid fat, sugar and alcohol.

Ingredient Benefit

Beetroot contains a powerful antioxidant betacyanin, which helps detoxification inside the liver.

Celery has diuretic properties and helps with toxic elimination. Decreases uric acid in the blood, which lowers the risk of getting kidney stones.

Apples contain antioxidants that prevent the growth of cancer cells in the bowel and liver.

Spinach, spirulina & chlorella contain chlorophyll which help the liver get rid of harmful dietary and environmental toxins.

Carrots contain sulphur and glutathione, which help the detoxification process in the liver.

Citrus fruit contains vitamin C which helps nullify and remove harmful toxins.

Green tea cold green tea contains catechins, powerful detoxifying antioxidant.

ANTI-AGEING SMOOTHIE INGREDIENTS

20g Cashew nuts

10g Sesame seeds

10g Sunflower seeds

50g Oats

20g Pumpkins seeds

Big handful of Spinach

20g Brazil nuts

50g Citrus fruits

Half an Avocado

Coconut water

METHOD

Add all of the ingredients to your mixer, top up with coconut water and blend.

AVOID

If you're worried about signs of ageing it's a good idea to generally avoid too much fructose (limit yourself to 2 pieces of fruit each day), low fat products and grains. Too many grains, such as rice and quinoa, can be harmful as they contain phytates, which bind on to essential nutrients such as zinc and manganese and prevent their absorption. These nutrients are needed to produce powerful antioxidants.

Ingredient Benefit

Cashews, sesame & sunflower seeds contain copper, which help produce a really powerful antioxidant called Superoxide Dismutase (SOD).

Oats & pumpkin seeds contain zinc, which also helps to produce SOD.

Spinach contains manganese, which again helps produce SOD.

Brazil nuts contain selenium, which is needed to produce glutathione peroxidase (GPx) another really important and powerful antioxidant needed in the body.

Citrus fruits contain antioxidants needed to eradicate free radicals. Free radicals speed up the ageing process. Antioxidants help quench those free radicals, thus slowing the ageing process.

Avocado contains powerful antioxidants like vitamin E.

Coconut water contains bioactive enzymes that aid digestion, is full of potassium and is also good for a bit of extra flavor

SKIN SMOOTHIE

INGREDIENTS

40g Red apple

40g Berries

15g Almonds

15g Cashews

Handful of Swiss chard

20g Brazil nuts

20g Goji berries

Coconut water

METHOD

Add all of the ingredients to your mixer, top up with coconut water and blend.

AVOID

If you suffer with skin issues it's a good idea to generally try and avoid low fat diets, artificial fats, grains and phytates.

Ingredient Benefit

Red berries & apple contain bioflavonoids and antioxidants, which reduce inflammation and protect cells.

Almonds, cashews & Swiss chard contain oxalic acid, which has been shown to clear skin of blemishes.

Brazil nuts contain selenium, which improves immune function and protects cells against damage. Selenium also promotes growth of hair and nails.

Goji berries help to repair skin damage.

Coconut water contains bioactive enzymes that aid digestion, is full of potassium and is also good for a bit of extra flavour.

BRAIN BOOSTING SMOOTHIE

INGREDIENTS

20g Sunflower seeds

HAndful of Spinach

50g Cantaloupe melon

HAndful of Kale

20g Almonds

20g Flax seeds

Half an Avocado

Coconut water

METHOD

Add all of the ingredients to your mixer, top up with coconut water and blend.

Ingredient Benefit

Sunflower seeds & spinach both contain B vitamins, which slow the rate of brain shrinkage and the onset of Alzheimer's.

Wheatbran, almonds & cashews contain magnesium, which helps to strengthen bones.

Cantaloupe melon, kale & almonds all contain vitamin E, which protects the brain against toxic protons, and are powerful anti-oxidants preventing build up of free radicals in the brain. They also contain vitamin A.

Flax seeds & avocado contain omega 3, which improves brain health.

Coconut water contains bioactive enzymes that aid digestion, is full of potassium and is also good for a bit of extra flavour.

MILDLY SPICED CHICKEN & RICE

CALORIES / MACRONUTRIENTS PER SERVING

Calories Protein Fat Carb

607 52g 24g 32g

METHOD

Saute the onion and garlic in a large frying pan for a couple of minutes and then add the red pepper, chicken thighs, the spices and some seasoning, the raw white rice, cherry tomatoes and chicken stock (enough to cover the rice). Bring to the boil and simmer for about 15 minutes until the chicken and rice are cooked through. Just before you take off the heat add the spinach for 1 minute, so it wilts nicely in the heat.

INGREDIENTS

Serves 2

1 Onion, finely chopped

2 Cloves of garlic, finely chopped

1 Red pepper, sliced

6 x Chicken thighs (skinless and boneless) cut into large pieces

2 tsp of curry or chilli powder

100g White rice

150g Cherry tomatoes, halved

500ml Chicken stock

100g Spinach

SPICY CHICKEN & BROWN RICE

CALORIES / MACRONUTRIENTS PER SERVING

Calories Protein Fat Carb

612   44g   17g 44g

METHOD

Skin and de-bone your chicken thighs, if not already done. Finely slice the onions. Measure and mix the spices before coating the chicken thighs with them. In a large saucepan that can go in the oven add the brown rice, the onion and garlic, chicken thighs, cherry tomatoes and hot chicken stock (you need enough stock to cover the rice and sit halfway up the chicken). Place the lid on top and place in the oven at 180 degrees until cooked through (45 min to an hour). Add the spinach right at the end and allow it to gently steam in the heat with the lid on. Garnish with coriander & enjoy!

INGREDIENTS

Serves 4

8 Chicken thighs (remove skin & bone, but keep whole)

1 Onion, finely sliced

1 tsp Cayenne pepper

1 tsp Sweet paprika

1 tsp Cumin

1 tsp Garam masala

1 tsp Cinnamon

1 tsp Turmeric

200g Brown rice

200g Cherry tomatoes, halved

400g Chick peas

500-750ml Hot chicken stock

100g Spinach

Coriander to garnish

9 798441 413121